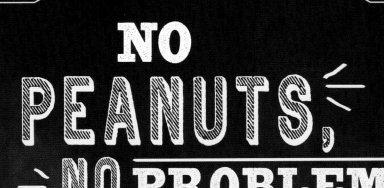

NO PEANUTS, NO PROBLEM!

Easy and Delicious Nut-free Recipes
for Kids With Allergies

by **KATRINA JORGENSEN**

CONSULTANT
Amy Durkan MS, RDN, CDN
Nutrition Research Manager
Mount Sinai Medical Center
New York, NY, USA

raintree
a Capstone company — publishers for children

Raintree is an imprint of Capstone Global Library Limited, a company incorporated in England and Wales having its registered office at 264 Banbury Road, Oxford, OX2 7DY – Registered company number: 6695582

www.raintree.co.uk
myorders@raintree.co.uk

Edited by Anna Butzer
Designed by Heidi Thompson
Picture research by Morgan Walters
Production by Kathy McColley

ISBN 978 1 4747 1068 8
20 19 18 17 16
10 9 8 7 6 5 4 3 2 1

British Library Cataloguing in Publication Data
A full catalogue record for this book is available from the British Library.

Every effort has been made to contact copyright holders of material reproduced in this book. Any omissions will be rectified in subsequent printings if notice is given to the publisher. All the internet addresses (URLs) given in this book were valid at the time of going to press. However, due to the dynamic nature of the internet, some addresses may have changed, or sites may have changed or ceased to exist since publication. While the author and publisher regret any inconvenience this may cause readers, no responsibility for any such changes can be accepted by either the author or the publisher.

Design Elements
Shutterstock: avian, design element, Katerina Kirilova, design element, Lena Pan, design element, Marco Govel, design element, mexrix, design element, Sabina Pittak, design element, STILLFX, design element, swatchandsoda, design element

Photography by Capstone Studio: Karon Dubke

Editor's note:
Capstone cannot ensure that any food is allergen-free. The only way to be sure a food is safe is to read all labels carefully, every time. Cross-contamination is also a risk for those with food allergies. Please phone food companies to make sure their manufacturing processes avoid cross-contamination. Also, always make sure you clean hands, surfaces and tools before cooking.

Printed in China.

CONTENTS

WHAT IS A FOOD ALLERGY?

Our bodies are armed with immune systems. It's the immune system's job to fight infections, viruses and invaders. Sometimes the immune system identifies a particular food as one of these invaders and attacks it. While our immune system fights, a chemical response is triggered and causes an allergic reaction. Reactions vary greatly from a mild skin irritation to having trouble breathing. Whenever you feel you are having a reaction, tell an adult immediately.

The best way to avoid having an allergic reaction is to be aware of what you are eating. Be careful not to consume that allergen. If you are not sure if that allergen is in a food, ask an adult or read the ingredients label of the food container before eating. Unfortunately, allergens can sometimes be hard to identify in an ingredient list. Have a look at www.allergyuk.org/peanut-and-tree-nut-allergy/peanut-and-tree-nut-allergy for a full list of which foods to avoid.

Avoiding food allergens can be hard to do, especially when they are found in so many of our favourite foods. This cookbook will take you on a culinary journey to explore many of the dishes you've had to avoid because of a peanut or tree nut allergy.

Kitchen safety

A safe kitchen is a fun kitchen! Always start your recipes with clean hands, surfaces and tools. Wash your hands and any tools you may use in future steps of a recipe, especially when handling raw meat. Make sure you have an adult nearby to help you with any task you don't feel comfortable doing, such as cutting vegetables or carrying hot pans.

ALLERGY ALERTS AND TIPS

Have other food allergies? No problem.
Have a look at the list at the end of each recipe
for substitutions for other common allergens.
Look out for other cool tips and ideas too!

CONVERSIONS

1/4 teaspoon	1.25 grams or millilitres
1/2 teaspoon	2.5 g or mL
1 teaspoon	5 g or mL
1 tablespoon	15 g or mL
10 grams	1/3 ounce
50 grams	1 3/4 oz
100 grams	3 1/2 oz
455 grams	16 oz (1 pound)
10 mL	1/3 fluid oz
50 mL	1 3/4 fl oz
100 mL	3 1/2 fl oz

Fahrenheit (°F)	Celsius (°C)
325°	160°
350°	180°
375°	190°
400°	200°
425°	220°
450°	230°

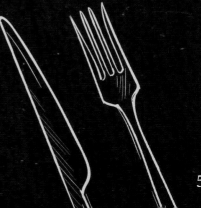

SESAME GRANOLA BARS

Get ready for granola on the go! Nuts are almost always found in granola, but you can make homemade bars that are nut free. Crunchy and delicious, these granola bars will satisfy your hunger when you're out and about.

Preparation time: 30 minutes (20 minutes inactive)

Cooking time: 15 minutes

Makes 12 bars

Ingredients

200 grams rolled oats

180 grams pitted dates

90 grams honey

60 grams sunflower seed butter

1 tablespoon tahini
  (sesame seed paste)

2 tablespoons sunflower seeds

2 tablespoons flax seeds

3 tablespoons sesame seeds

Tools

large baking tray

measuring spoons/scales

food processor

large mixing bowl

20 x 20-centimetre (8 x 8-inch)
  baking dish

baking parchment

chef's knife

Allergen alert!

Many dates and dried fruits
are manufactured with nuts.
Check labels carefully, and call
the manufacturer for details.

Make sure your rolled oats are certified
wheat free if you avoid wheat.

1. Preheat oven to 180°C. Evenly spread out the rolled oats on a large baking tray. Place in the oven for 15 minutes, or until golden brown.

2. While the oats bake, place the dates in the food processor. Blend on high until the dates look like a ball of dough. Add the honey, sunflower seed butter and tahini, and pulse until well blended.

3. Place the toasted oats and all seeds in the large bowl. Carefully remove the blade from the food processor and pour in the date mixture.

4. Use your hands to squish the mixture until the oats and seeds are coated well.

5. Wash your hands. Line the bottom of the baking dish with baking parchment.

6. Empty the contents of the mixing bowl into the baking dish. Use your hands to press the mixture flat, making one large square.

7. Place the dish in a refrigerator for at least 20 minutes to harden.

8. Slice into 12 bars.

9. Wrap in baking parchment and keep in the refrigerator for up to one week.

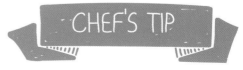

CHEF'S TIP

Keep your bars for a longer period of time
by placing them in your freezer. Put one in
your lunchbox in the morning and it will be
perfectly thawed for your midday meal!

APPLE MUFFINS

Grab the muffin tin and get ready to bake! These sweet treats are a perfect nut-free addition to the breakfast table. You'll fall in love with these fluffy muffins overflowing with flavour!

Preparation time: 15 minutes

Cooking time: 30 minutes

Makes 12 muffins

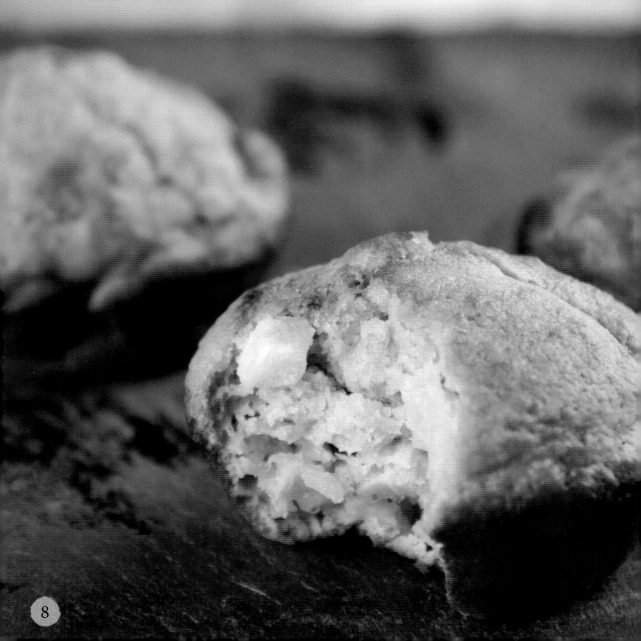

Ingredients

2 tablespoons milled flaxseed

60 millilitres water

1 Granny Smith apple

250 grams plain flour

100 grams caster sugar

1½ tablespoons pumpkin pie spice

1 teaspoon bicarbonate of soda

1 teaspoon baking powder

370 grams apple sauce

125 millilitres sunflower oil

Tools

standard muffin tin

12 muffin cases

measuring spoons/scales/jug

2 mixing bowls

whisk

peeler

chopping board

chef's knife

spoon

toothpick

Allergen alert!

If you're avoiding wheat, make sure
you use wheat-free flour
instead of plain flour.

1. Preheat oven to 180°C. Line muffin tin with cases and set aside.

2. In a mixing bowl, combine the milled flaxseed and water. Stir with a whisk. Allow to sit for at least five minutes.

3. Peel and core the apple, and then cut into small cubes. Set aside.

4. In the unused mixing bowl, add the remaining dry ingredients. Stir to combine.

5. Add apple sauce and sunflower oil to the flaxseed mix. Whisk to combine, then pour over the flour mixture.

6. Stir until most lumps are gone.

7. Drop in the apples. Stir until coated.

8. Fill each of the muffin cups two-thirds full.

9. Place in the oven for about 30 minutes. Insert a toothpick in the centre of a muffin. If it comes out clean, the muffins are done. Remove muffins from the oven and allow to cool slightly before serving.

10. Store leftovers in an airtight container at room temperature for up to one week.

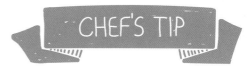

CHEF'S TIP

Want to add another flavour into the mix?
Swap the apple sauce for 370 grams
pumpkin puree.

BANANA-CHOCOLATE CRÈME
PANCAKES

Bananas + chocolate = YUM! Hazelnuts are an ingredient in chocolate crème, but you can get the same taste and texture with sunflower seed butter. Whip up a sweet pancake breakfast that your family will love!

Preparation time: 10 minutes

Cooking time: 10 minutes

Makes 8–10 pancakes

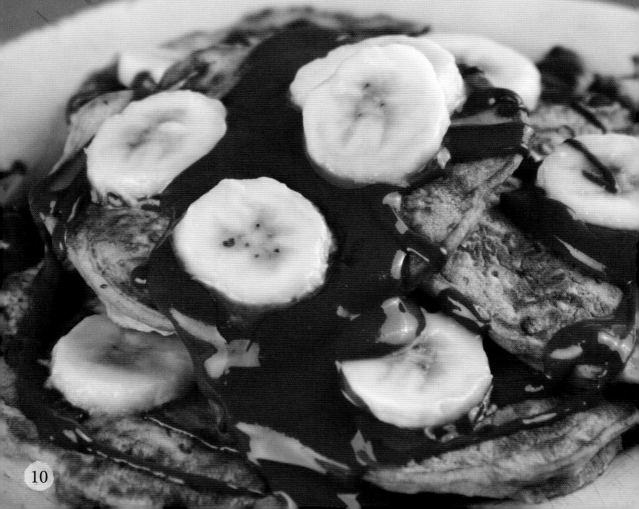

Ingredients

Chocolate crème

125 grams sunflower seed butter

2 tablespoons cocoa powder

2 tablespoons honey

Banana pancakes

3 bananas

180 grams plain flour

240 millilitres water

1 teaspoon baking powder

¼ teaspoon salt

cooking spray

Tools

2 mixing bowls

measuring spoons/scales/jug

2 forks

chef's knife

chopping board

whisk

frying pan

ladle

spatula

Allergen alert!

Cocoa and chocolate are often manufactured with nuts. Check labels carefully, and call the manufacturer for details.

Replace the plain flour with wheat-free flour if you're avoiding wheat!

1. In a mixing bowl, combine all crème ingredients. Mix well with a fork. Set aside.

2. Peel the bananas, and slice two of them into 1.3-centimetre (½-inch) rounds. Set aside. Mash the last banana well with a fork.

3. Scrape the mashed banana into a second mixing bowl. Add the flour, water, baking powder and salt. Whisk until most lumps are gone.

4. Place the frying pan on the hob on medium heat.

5. When the pan is hot, add cooking spray to the surface. Then scoop 120 millilitres of batter onto the hot pan.

6. Allow to cook until bubbles appear around the edges.

7. Using the spatula, flip the pancake. Cook until golden brown.

8. Remove the pancake from the heat and place on a plate. Repeat steps 5 to 8 until all batter is gone.

9. To serve, spread 2 tablespoons of the chocolate crème on a pancake, followed by 6–7 slices of banana.

10. Serve immediately. Leftover chocolate crème can be stored in the refrigerator for up to two weeks.

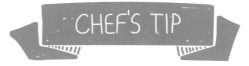

CHEF'S TIP

Don't want to monkey around with bananas? Slice up 225 grams of strawberries instead for a sweet alternative!

APPLE **SANDWICH**

Make your own sandwich – without bread or peanut butter! Cast aside the bread and use apples instead. Sunflower seed butter takes over the role of peanut butter so you can be nut-free without sacrificing the flavour.

Preparation time: 5 minutes

Cooking time: 1 minute

Makes 2 apple sandwiches

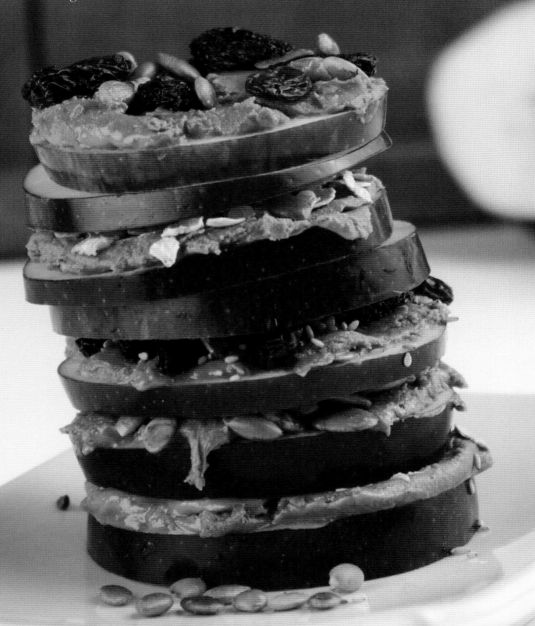

Ingredients

1 apple — your favourite kind

1 lemon

4 tablespoons sunflower seed butter

2 tablespoons of your choice of topping:
rolled oats, raisins, pumpkin seeds,
sesame seeds or jam

Tools

chopping board

chef's knife

small round biscuit cutter

measuring spoons

butter knife

---

1. Carefully cut the top and bottom off the apple, about 1.3-centimetre (½-inch) thick. Enjoy those pieces later!

2. Cut the remaining apple into four even slices for making two sandwiches. Set aside.

3. Using the round biscuit cutter, cut the cores out of each slice and discard.

4. Cut the lemon in half. Gently squeeze a few drops of juice on both sides of the apple slices.

5. Spread 2 tablespoons of sunflower seed butter on two of the apple slices.

6. Sprinkle or spread your choice of topping over the sunflower seed butter.

7. Place the plain apple slices over the sunflower seed butter slices to make a sandwich.

8. Eat immediately, or store in an airtight container for up to one day.

Allergen alert!

Dried fruits, such as raisins and seeds, are often manufactured with nuts. Check labels carefully, and call the manufacturer for details.

If you're going to put rolled oats on your sandwich, make sure you get a wheat-free version if you're avoiding wheat.

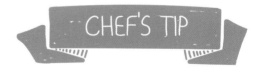

CHEF'S TIP

Why put lemon on your apples? When you slice an apple, you expose the pulp to oxygen that causes it to turn brown. It's OK to eat apple slices that have turned brown (within a day or two of slicing). The acid in lemon juice forms a protective barrier that keeps your apples looking perfectly fresh!

THAI CHICKEN SALAD

How do you get a nutty flavour without the nuts? With sesame seeds! Peanuts are a staple ingredient in Thai food, but you won't miss them in this crunchy salad topped with a tangy dressing.

Preparation time: 20 minutes

Cooking time: 15 minutes

Serves 4

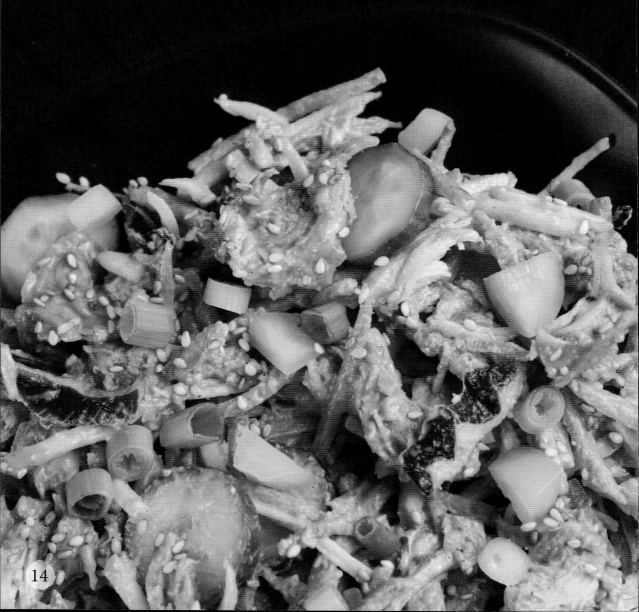

Ingredients

Dressing

60 grams sunflower seed butter

2 teaspoons tahini
  (sesame seed paste)

2 tablespoons lime juice

3 tablespoons olive oil

1 tablespoon coconut aminos

3 tablespoons honey

1 tablespoon crushed garlic

1 tablespoon crushed ginger

½ teaspoon salt

handful fresh coriander leaves

Salad

455 grams boneless, skinless
  chicken thighs

1 teaspoon salt

½ teaspoon pepper

2 tablespoons olive oil

1 bell pepper

1 cucumber

400 grams coleslaw mix

1 spring onion

2 teaspoons sesame seeds

Tools

blender

measuring spoons/scales

chopping board

chef's knife

frying pan

serving bowl

tongs

1. In a blender, combine all of the dressing ingredients. Blend on high until smooth.

2. Cut the chicken into bite-sized pieces. Sprinkle with salt and pepper.

3. Wash your hands, chopping board and chef's knife after you have finished handling the chicken.

4. Heat the olive oil in a frying pan over medium-high heat and add the chicken.

5. Cook the chicken on all sides, about eight to 10 minutes, or until no longer pink in the centre. Set aside.

6. Cut the stem off the bell pepper, and then cut down the centre. Carefully pull out the seeds and discard. Cut the pepper into small pieces and set aside.

7. Slice the cucumber into 0.6-centimetre (¼-inch) rounds and set aside.

8. To assemble the salad, place the coleslaw mix, bell pepper, cucumber and chicken in a serving bowl.

9. Drizzle half of the dressing over the salad. Toss with tongs to coat all of the ingredients.

10. Add more dressing if necessary, then sprinkle with sesame seeds.

11. Serve immediately with leftover dressing on the side, if desired.

Allergen alert!

Although sesame isn't considered one of the top eight food allergens, it's a very common allergy. Leave the sesame seeds off if you're allergic to them.

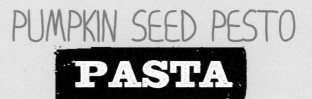

PUMPKIN SEED PESTO
PASTA

You may get tongue-tied trying to say this recipe name, but you can reward your taste buds with this light and fresh pasta. Pesto is usually made with pine nuts, but pumpkin seeds allow you to keep nuts out of the recipe.

Preparation time: 5 minutes

Cooking time: 15 minutes

Serves 4

Ingredients

3.75 litres water

2 tablespoons salt

225 grams pasta, any shape

Pesto

3 handfuls fresh basil leaves

60 millilitres extra virgin olive oil

30 grams pumpkin seeds

2 garlic cloves

½ teaspoon lemon juice

25 grams shredded Parmesan cheese

½ teaspoon salt

¼ teaspoon ground black pepper

Tools

large saucepan

measuring spoons/scales/jug

blender

colander

serving bowl

tongs

1. Place water in a large saucepan with salt. Place pan on the hob on high.

2. When the water begins to boil, add the pasta. Reduce heat to a low boil. Cook according to package directions.

3. Combine all pesto ingredients in a blender. Blend on high until smooth. Set aside.

4. When the pasta is cooked, carefully drain into a colander.

5. Transfer pasta to a serving bowl and add half of the pesto.

6. Toss gently with tongs until the pasta is coated. Add more pesto if desired.

7. Serve immediately. Store leftover pesto in an airtight container in a refrigerator for up to three days.

Allergen alert!

Do you need to avoid dairy? Trade the Parmesan cheese for equal parts nutritional yeast.

Egg-free or wheat-free pasta can be used in place of normal pasta.

HONEY GARLIC
CHICKEN WINGS

Want something finger-lickin' good but also easy to make? These sticky and sweet glazed chicken wings are sure to please. Whether you're serving them for a jazzed-up weeknight meal or a tantalizing party appetizer, these crispy wings with bold flavour will be the star!

Preparation time: 15 minutes

Cooking time: 2 hours 40 minutes
  (2½ hours inactive)

Serves 4 as a meal, 8 as an appetizer

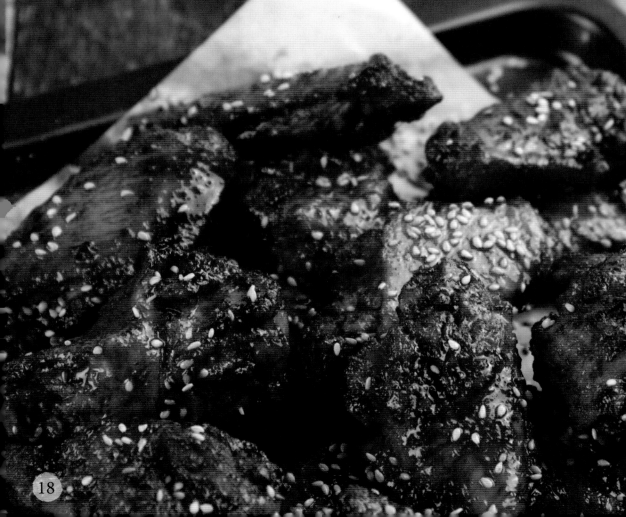

Ingredients

2 tablespoons crushed garlic

60 millilitres olive oil

85 grams honey

2 tablespoons soya sauce

2 tablespoons brown sugar

1 teaspoon cornflour

910 grams bone-in chicken wings
(about 24 wings)

1 teaspoon salt

½ teaspoon black pepper

1 tablespoon sesame seeds

Tools

measuring spoons/scales/jug

medium mixing bowl

whisk

chopping board

kitchen roll

tongs

3 litre slow cooker

large baking tray

baking parchment

ladle

Allergen alert!

If you're allergic to soya, you can
use an equal amount of coconut aminos
instead of soya sauce.

Leave the sesame seeds off
if you have a sesame allergy.

1. Combine the first six ingredients in a medium mixing bowl. Whisk until smooth. Set aside.

2. Place the chicken wings on a chopping board and pat dry with kitchen roll.

3. Sprinkle salt and pepper on both sides of the wings. Pat with hands to make sure it sticks. Wash your hands when finished.

4. Use tongs to place the wings in the bottom of the slow cooker. Pour sauce over top. Stir to coat.

5. Put the lid on the slow cooker and set on high for two and a half hours.

6. When the wings are almost done, preheat oven to 230°C. Line a large baking tray with baking parchment and set aside.

7. When the wings are done, use tongs to place them on the baking tray about 1.3 centimetres (½ inch) apart.

8. Place in the oven for about 10 minutes, or until the skin is slightly crispy and browned.

9. Ladle the remaining sauce over the wings. Toss to coat.

10. Sprinkle with sesame seeds and serve hot.

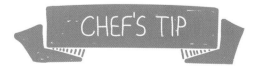

CHEF'S TIP

You don't want to use chicken wings? You can make
this recipe with chicken thighs or drumsticks. Just
add an hour of cooking time to your slow cooker
(3½ hours, instead of 2½).

19

SESAME GREEN
BEANS

Add some flair to the dinner table with Asian-inspired green beans. A play on green beans almondine, this dish replaces almonds with sesame seeds for a delicious crunch.

Preparation time: 5 minutes

Cooking time: 5 minutes

Serves 4

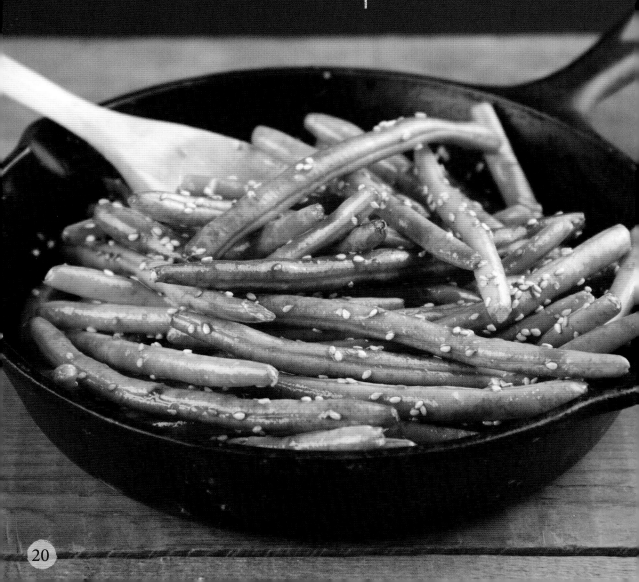

Ingredients

455 grams fresh green beans

2 teaspoons olive oil

1 teaspoon toasted sesame oil

1 teaspoon coconut aminos

1 teaspoon honey

1 tablespoon sesame seeds

Tools

measuring spoons

frying pan

tongs

wooden spoon

serving bowl

Allergen alert!

You can leave the sesame seeds off
if you have a sesame allergy.

1. Cook green beans in the microwave according to directions on package. Set aside to cool slightly.

2. In a frying pan, heat the olive oil over medium-high heat.

3. Carefully uncover the beans. Watch out for hot steam. Pour the green beans into the frying pan.

4. Using tongs, toss the green beans around to coat with oil.

5. Add the sesame oil, coconut aminos and honey.

6. Stir the green beans quickly as the sauce begins to slightly thicken.

7. Transfer the green beans to a serving bowl. Sprinkle with sesame seeds.

8. Toss gently with tongs to coat all of the beans. Serve hot.

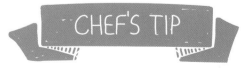

CHEF'S TIP

You can use any green vegetable you like
for this recipe, such as broccoli, spinach,
peas or asparagus!

BBQ ROASTED
CHICKPEAS

Combine a smoky BBQ flavour with the crunch of roasted chickpeas and you get a tasty snack! These chickpeas are not only delicious but they are also a healthy treat loaded with protein.

Preparation time: 40 minutes (30 minutes inactive)

Cooking time: 45 minutes

Makes 4 servings

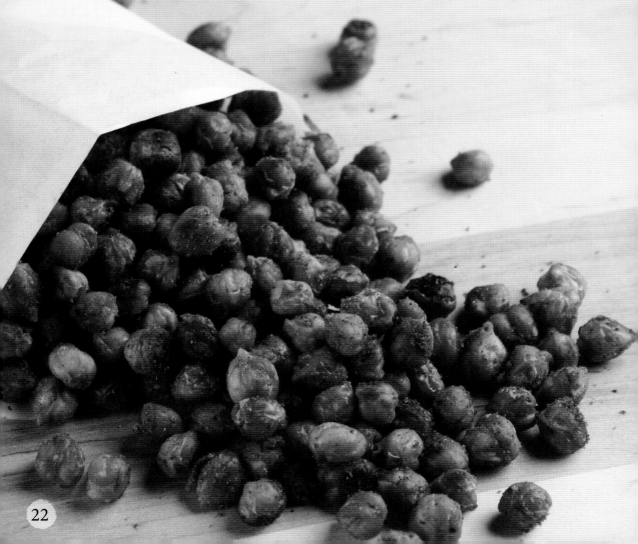

Ingredients

850 grams chickpeas

2 teaspoons brown sugar

2 teaspoons salt

2 teaspoons garlic powder

½ teaspoon ground white pepper

1 teaspoon dry mustard

½ teaspoon cayenne pepper

½ teaspoon cumin

2 teaspoons smoked paprika

2 tablespoons olive oil

Tools

baking tray

baking parchment

can opener

colander

kitchen roll

mixing bowl

measuring spoons

spatula

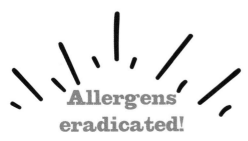

Allergens eradicated!

No major food allergens found here!

1. Preheat oven to 200°C. Line a baking tray with baking parchment and set aside.

2. Open the tins of chickpeas and empty them into the colander.

3. Keeping the chickpeas in the colander, rinse with cool water.

4. Line a clean surface with kitchen roll and spread the chickpeas on top.

5. Allow to sit for about 30 minutes to dry almost completely.

6. While the chickpeas dry, make your flavouring. Combine remaining ingredients in a mixing bowl. Stir until smooth.

7. When the chickpeas are mostly dry, transfer them to the mixing bowl. Stir to coat evenly.

8. Spread the chickpeas evenly on the baking tray.

9. Bake in the oven for about 45 minutes, or until golden brown and hardened.

10. Remove from oven and allow to cool slightly before serving.

11. Store leftovers in an airtight container for up to three days.

SUNFLOWER SEED BUTTER
COOKIES

With the help of sunflower seed butter, you can make a nut-free dessert with a nutty flavour! Crunchy on the outside and soft on the inside, these simple cookies are made with only five ingredients.

Preparation time: 10 minutes

Cooking time: 10 minutes

Makes 12 cookies

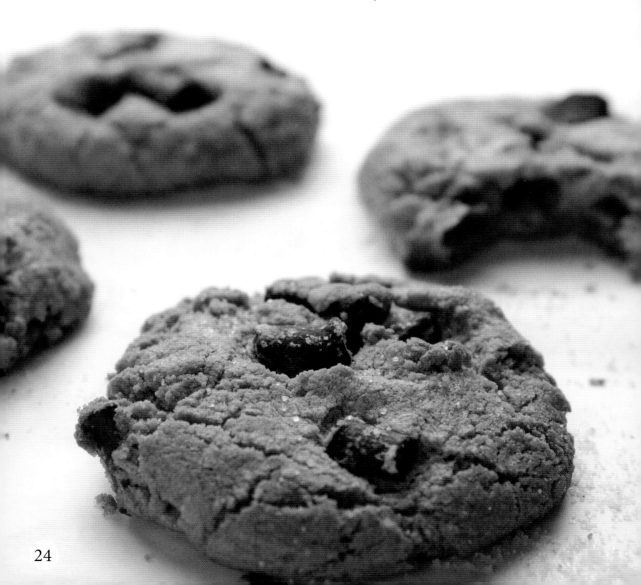

Ingredients

2 tablespoons milled flaxseed

60 millilitres water

250 grams sunflower seed butter

150 grams caster sugar

50 grams brown sugar

Tools

baking tray

baking parchment

measuring spoons/scales/jug

mixing bowl

spatula

cooling rack

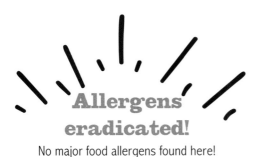

Allergens eradicated!

No major food allergens found here!

1. Preheat the oven to 180°C. Line a baking tray with baking parchment.

2. In a mixing bowl, combine the milled flaxseed and water. Stir and allow to sit for five minutes before continuing.

3. Add the sunflower seed butter, sugar and brown sugar to the flaxseed mixture. Stir well until it begins to thicken, about one minute.

4. Divide the dough into 12 equally sized pieces. Roll into balls between your palms.

5. Place the dough balls on the baking tray, evenly spaced. Leave at least 5 centimetres (2 inches) of space between the balls.

6. Use your palm to flatten each dough ball slightly.

7. Place in the oven and bake for about 10 minutes.

8. Remove from oven and allow to cool for five minutes before transferring to a cooling rack.

9. Serve warm or at room temperature and store leftovers in an airtight container for up to three days.

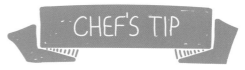

CHEF'S TIP

Are you craving chocolate? Add chocolate chips to the mix in step 3! Make sure the chocolate chips you use are free of allergens.

CHOCOLATE SUNFLOWER
CUPS

Give the American-style peanut butter cup a nut-free makeover! Delight your taste buds by combining smooth milk chocolate and creamy sunflower seed butter into one delectable, bite-sized dessert.

Preparation time: 1 hour 10 minutes (1 hour inactive)

Makes 12 cups

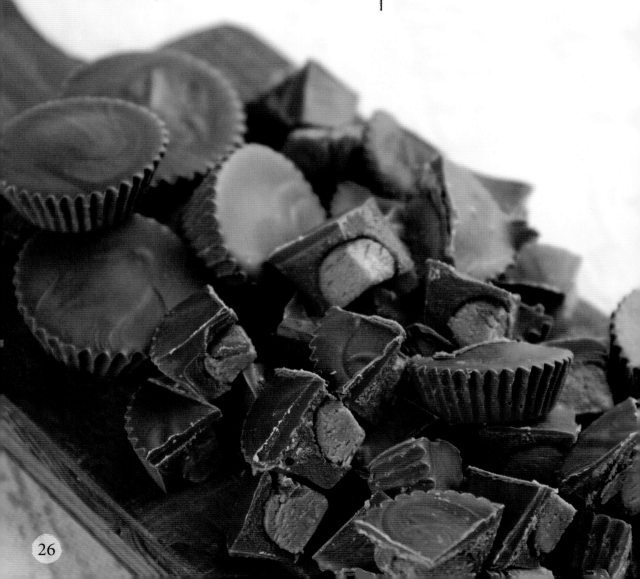

Ingredients

cooking spray

125 grams sunflower seed butter

30 grams icing sugar

¼ teaspoon salt

175 grams chocolate chips

Tools

mini muffin tin

12 mini muffin cases

mixing bowl

measuring spoons/scales

spatula

microwave-safe bowl

Allergen alert!

Chocolate chips can contain or be manufactured with soya, nuts and dairy. Make sure you check that the chocolate chips you use are free of allergens.

1. Place 12 mini muffin cases in a mini muffin tin. Spray a small amount of cooking spray in each case and set aside.

2. In a mixing bowl, combine the sunflower seed butter, icing sugar and salt. Mix until thickened. Add more icing sugar if needed.

3. Divide the dough into 12 pieces. Roll each piece between your palms to make 12 small balls. Set aside.

4. In a microwave-safe bowl, melt the chocolate chips by cooking on medium for two minutes. Stir, and then cook on medium an additional minute.

5. To assemble, spread a small amount of chocolate in each case, followed by a sunflower seed butter ball. Top with remaining chocolate, until the ball is covered.

6. Place in refrigerator to cool for at least one hour.

7. Store leftovers in refrigerator for up to one week, or in freezer for up to one month.

NO-NUT
BRITTLE

What do you get when you take the peanuts out of peanut brittle? No-nut brittle! Pumpkin seeds add to the crunch in this caramel-flavoured sweet.

Preparation time: 10 minutes

Cooking time: 2½ hours
  (2 hours inactive)

Serves 10–12

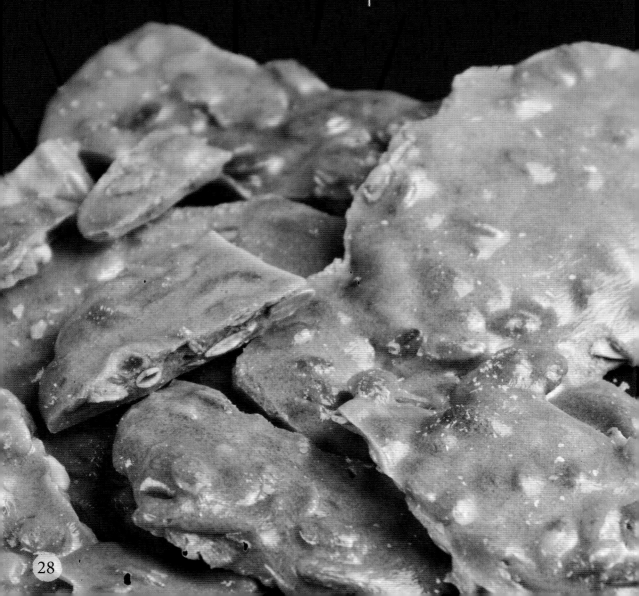

Ingredients

100 grams granulated sugar

100 grams brown sugar

115 grams corn syrup

130 grams pumpkin seeds

1 teaspoon butter

½ teaspoon vanilla extract

½ teaspoon maple extract

1 teaspoon bicarbonate of soda

Tools

20 x 20-cm (8 x 8-in) baking dish

baking parchment

measuring spoons/scales

large microwave-safe mixing bowl

spatula

Allergen alert!

Butter can be replaced with a
dairy-free butter in this recipe for
those who are avoiding dairy.

1. Line a baking dish with baking parchment and set aside.

2. In a mixing bowl, combine the granulated sugar, brown sugar and corn syrup. Microwave on high for three minutes.

3. Carefully remove from microwave and add the pumpkin seeds. Stir to combine.

4. Return bowl to microwave and cook on high for an additional three minutes.

5. Remove bowl from the microwave. Add the butter, vanilla extract and maple extract. Stir carefully.

6. Microwave on high for one minute.

7. Remove from microwave and add the bicarbonate of soda. Stir to combine.

8. Pour into prepared baking dish, and allow to sit for at least two hours to cool.

9. When cooled, break into pieces for serving.

10. Store leftovers in an airtight container at room temperature for up to one week.

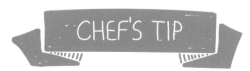

CHEF'S TIP

Don't mess with the crunch! Replace
pumpkin seeds with other seeds such
as sesame or sunflower seeds.

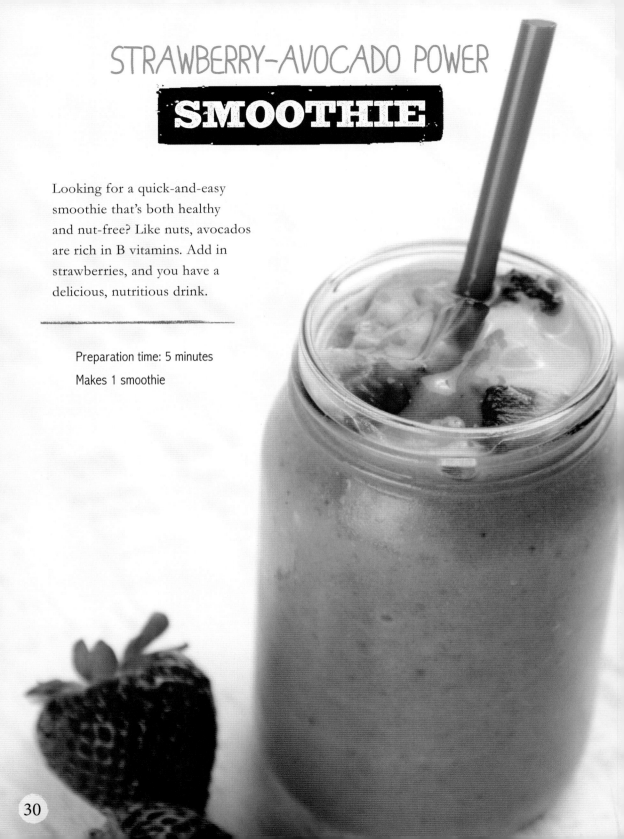

STRAWBERRY-AVOCADO POWER

SMOOTHIE

Looking for a quick-and-easy
smoothie that's both healthy
and nut-free? Like nuts, avocados
are rich in B vitamins. Add in
strawberries, and you have a
delicious, nutritious drink.

Preparation time: 5 minutes

Makes 1 smoothie

Ingredients

½ avocado

75 grams frozen strawberries

1 frozen banana

120 millilitres milk

1 tablespoon honey

Tools

chopping board

chef's knife

spoon

measuring spoons/scales/jug

blender

Allergen alert!

Make sure you select a milk
that meets your dietary needs,
or use your favourite fruit juice.

1. Carefully slice the avocado in half and remove the pit.

2. Scoop half of the avocado flesh into the blender, followed by the frozen strawberries, banana, milk and honey.

3. Blend on high until smooth.

4. Pour into a serving glass, and serve immediately with a large straw.

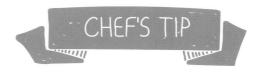

CHEF'S TIP

Wishing for a thicker smoothie? Add a handful of
crushed ice to your blender for a triple-thick delight!

Freezing your own fruit is fast and easy.

Strawberries: Wash and dry the strawberries well.
Cut the stems off the tops of the strawberries,
then slice each lengthwise.

Bananas: Peel the bananas and
slice them into 1.3-centimetre (½-inch) rounds.

To freeze your fruits: Line a baking tray
with baking parchment and place strawberries
and banana slices on it, flat sides down.
Freeze for three hours and then transfer to
a freezer-safe resealable bag.

GLOSSARY

assemble put all the parts of something together

blend mix together, sometimes using a blender

boil heat until large bubbles form on top of a liquid;
the boiling point for water is 100°C (212°F)

consume eat or drink something

discard throw something away because it is not needed

drizzle let a substance fall in small drops

mash smash a soft food into a lumpy mixture

pit single central seed or stone of some fruits

pulp soft juicy or fleshy part of a fruit or vegetable

slice cut into thin pieces with a knife

thaw bring frozen food to room temperature

whisk stir a mixture rapidly until it's smooth

READ MORE

Allergy-free Cooking for Kids, Pamela Clark (Sterling Epicure, 2014

The Allergy-Free Family Cookbook, Fiona Heggie and Ellie Lux (Orion, 2015)

The Kids Only Cookbook, Sue Quinn (Quadrille Publishing, 2013)

WEBSITE

www.allergyuk.org

If you have any allergies, this is the website to go to. It provides lots of useful information and a helpline.